From Vulnerable to
Empowered

Transforming your Medical Health
and Doctor Experience

WILLIAM H EAGLSTEIN, MD

From Vulnerable to Empowered
© 2024 by William H Eaglstein, MD

ISBN: 979-8-3208-8525-4

CONTENTS

Acknowledgements v

Preface vii

Chapter 1: What Are Doctors? 1

Chapter 2: What is Expected from and by Doctors 7

Chapter 3: Generalists and Specialists 11

Chapter 4: Consultants, Experts, Specialists,
and Generalists 17

Chapter 5: Surgeons (Surgeon Doctors) 23

Chapter 6: Doctors and Therapy 27

Chapter 7: Doctors, Decisions, and Data 35

Chapter 8: Cosmetic Surgery and Cosmetic
Medicine 39

Chapter 9: Public Health Doctors and
Public Health 43

Chapter 10: Doctor's Dress 45

Chapter 11: Doctors, Extra Smart Patients,
Relatives and Friends, and
Concierge Medicine 47

Chapter 12: Doctor-Patient Relationship 51

Chapter 13: Who Become Doctors................................55

Chapter 14: Physician Assistants 61

Chapter 15: The Medical Environment in the
United States...65

Chapter 16: Some Other Considerations 71

ACKNOWLEDGEMENTS

I thank my wife, Janet, for arranging our lives to allow me to pursue this and other works. Her editing skills are also much appreciated. Many thanks also to Professor William M. Mason, whose scrutiny and insightful comments on the entire project were extremely helpful. Rick Markoff offered tremendous marketing research, significant critique and editing assistance. Judy Markoff's gifted assistance with cover designs was invaluable as was Teddy Shalon's who pushed me to think more deeply about presenting this work to the world. And the insights offered by Gordon and Colleen Strickland, Bruce Anderson, Eileen Cohen, Dr. Mark Cohen and Dr. Robert DeBusk are much appreciated.

PREFACE

I was prompted to write this booklet about doctors because of the puzzlements and questions regarding doctors I have heard from many friends and acquaintances. Their confusion and misunderstandings have been especially striking because some are adults and seniors who have had considerable exposure to doctors and the associated facilities and systems because of their age and infirmities. Upon reflection, this may not be quite so unexpected. As children, we are exposed to doctors by our parents or other adults with only the most superficial explanations of doctors' roles. As teens and young adults and even adults, except during pregnancy, childbirth, and traumatic accidents, most people only rarely have the need of "seeing the doctor." Other than those trained in the healing arts or in the associated support services, there may be no occasion for most people to be formally taught about what doctors are supposed to do, how they go about doing it, and the legal and societal framework in which they work. With that in mind, this booklet should be of interest to many now requiring frequent health care or helping someone else who requires frequent health care, those first entering their senior decades, and others, for example, people considering a career in the health sciences, who want help in understanding their potential career selection.

This booklet is aimed at broadly describing what doctors are charged with doing, how they are trained, how they think about and implement their skills, the social and legal context in which they operate, and many of the special words used to convey their roles to the public. The information is about doctors and care systems in the United States, but much of it is also applicable to Europe, Britain, Australia, Japan, and other advanced, Western-oriented societies. This information is put forward as a basis that will allow readers to better understand their place in the health-care matrix in order to judge the activities of their doctors and their options. This includes recognizing when and possibly which type of significant change is likely to result in better care.

The booklet begins with an overview of doctors, including the different types of doctors currently practicing in the Western world. Subsequent chapters will help readers understand the role of generalists, specialists, and consultants as well as how surgeons differ and how doctors who practice public health or cosmetic medicine have different but well-defined roles. How doctors think about therapy and make decisions is described, as are important ancillary areas such as the role of doctor assistants. The social and legal circumstances of doctors are discussed in many chapters, especially in the chapter about the doctor-patient relationship. Although not a major focus, the medical environment in the US has its own chapter. Issues such as selecting your doctor, foreign medical graduates, teaching hospitals and understanding your doctor are parts of the final chapter. Each chapter starts with one or two questions aimed at prompting consideration of issues or information in the chapter. Importantly, the chapters are not dependent upon each other and may be read in any order. In fact, I suggest that readers not read the chapters in sequence or try to read the book in its entirety over a short period of time, but that they first read the chapters which seem to interest them or relate best to current or past personal experience. Also, perhaps unexpectedly, is the generous use of quotes, anecdotes, and jokes throughout. Not only do they entertain, but they also serve as a shortcut into the mind for the kernels of truth embedded in them.

This booklet does not offer judgments on the current "systems" or proposals for improving current circumstances. Rather, the aim of this publication is to impart a formal understanding of doctors who are the key element in how most of us receive our medical care.

Some readers might find the narrow focus frustrating because they will inevitably have faced circumstances where some "simple" provision, alteration, improvement, or rethinking might have improved a past or even current experience. Regarding this frustration, my hope is that the grounding provided by the information in this publication will help readers to better their care and pursue information about their own specific issues and concerns in a deeper, more meaningful, and more effective fashion.

CHAPTER 1

WHAT ARE DOCTORS?

*In nothing do men more nearly approach the gods
than in giving health to men. — Cicero*

*Isn't it a bit unnerving that doctors call what
they do "practice"? — George Carlin*

What is a "learned intermediary"?

**What is the theory of medications offered by
homeopathic doctors?**

Given the explosion of information about health and
disease available to the public and the newly available
health-related technologies available for people to use,
the question of the doctor being replaced by some
combination of artificial intelligence and self-treatment
or treatment by lay people is often posed. That is, might
doctors someday soon be replaced by technology? This

question is best answered by understanding the phrase "learned intermediary."

In legal parlance, the learned intermediary doctrine has a narrow definition indicating that makers of therapeutic drugs are responsible for informing doctors rather than patients about a drug's actions, side effects, contraindications, interactions with other drugs, and so forth. The doctors, as "learned intermediaries," are responsible for informing patients and prescribing the drugs in such a way as to best obtain the desired effects and avoid undesired effects. The doctor's responsibility as a learned intermediary for drugs remains today, even in the United States which is one of only two countries where drug companies are allowed to advertise directly to the public. However, broadly speaking, doctors are and always have been learned intermediaries or appliers of technologies and theories to the treatment of patients. Understanding that we are all to some degree unique by the circumstances of our genetics, our living conditions, and our behaviors, there will always be a need for a translation or application of basic science and health information to specific persons and to specific circumstances. Artificial intelligence and associated technologies will ultimately still need to be applied to treating and advising individuals by those who understand both the technologies and the patients as well as their circumstances. Diagnosis and treatment options will be improved by artificial intelligence, as they have been by other technologies, but doctors will still be needed to add the human note, providing care that resonates with a given patient's needs.

Doctors are members of the so-called learned professions—clergy, law, and medicine. For most of history, medicine and the spiritual were embodied in the same person. However, in most of the world, these two roles have been separated. Today's doctors play a largely secular role and are licensed by governments. In the United States, the individual state governments license or allow doctors to restore, maintain, and promote health by studying, diagnosing, and treating disease or disease-related circumstances.

Strictly speaking, a "doctor" is someone who has earned a doctorate degree, that is, someone who has earned or been awarded the highest possible educational level offered by a university or college—for example, a doctor of history or law. In the United States, doctors of medicine have had four years of medical school training after their undergraduate training. Even after being awarded a doctorate in medicine, they often have many years of additional training and practice after medical school. The word "physician" indicates a medical doctor—so all physicians are doctors, but not all doctors are physicians.

Confusingly in the United States, there are several large categories of physicians: allopathic, osteopathic, and chiropractic. Although not generally used by the mainstream medical community in the United States, the term *allopath* has been used to describe traditional medical doctors. The term *allopathic* refers to using means such as medicine to induce effects opposite to the patient's symptom—for example, to reduce inflammation in inflammatory diseases. Allopathic medical doctors in the United States use the name suffix MD (medical doctors).

In contrast to MDs, osteopathic doctors or osteopaths use the suffix DO (doctors of osteopathy). This designation derives from their field's original belief that disease was related to a misalignment of the body's bones. Osteopathic and allopathic doctors now have largely similar and scientifically based training but in separate institutions. About 25 percent of medical students in the United States are in osteopathic medical schools. Chiropractic doctors or *chiropaths* emphasize the treatment of musculoskeletal problems and rely on physical and manipulative methods more than drug or surgical approaches.

Allopathic, osteopathic, and chiropractic doctors are licensed to practice in all US states and territories and many other countries.

The licensing process and the regulatory activities of each group are governed by state laws but executed by licensing bodies or medical boards. The medical boards are charged with protecting the public, and this is often done by requiring doctors to take additional or specific training. However, on occasion, medical boards revoke a physician's license to practice in order to protect the public. Generally, medical boards are composed of both physicians and members of the public. Most often, members are appointed by the governor of the state, but this varies by state.

Homeopathic and naturopathic doctors are common in Europe and India but can also be found in the US and many other countries. Their practice is based on a set of assumptions not consistent with the research underlying Western or mainstream medicine. One defining principle of homeopathy is that "like treats like." That is, homeopathic doctors treat with minuscule amounts of agents that cause the same symptoms the patient has with the idea of inducing a tolerance or a kind of immunization against the disease or its symptoms. This is in contrast with the allopathic idea of using agents that combat the patient's symptoms and disease. Depending upon the U.S. state, homeopaths may be overseen by a specific regulatory body.

A friend of mine was destined to be an osteopath.
He said he could feel it in his bones—

https://twitter.com/punsandoneliner/status/1716650730491433050 2/19/24

CHAPTER 2

WHAT IS EXPECTED FROM
AND BY DOCTORS

What are some of the standards that doctors are held to by law, custom, and oath?

Doctors like to be and are accorded the role of the good guys. Although doctors no longer aspire to and are no longer expected to assume priestly duties, they are generally accorded considerable respect, which in some cases can even border on reverence.

The special role given to doctors derives from many factors, including the physical intimacy associated with a doctor's examinations. Of course, patients understand that it is in their self-interest to overcome their modesty and allow doctors to examine even their most intimate areas. Parenthetically, in China and other parts of Asia, until recently, doctors, who were almost all male at the time, were not allowed to physically examine female patients. Rather, doctors had "doctor's dolls," (See Fig) which were reclining nude female dolls. Patients or their relatives pointed to the place on the doll where the patient had signs or symptoms. Today at medical visits in much of the world, patients not only overcome their own physical modesty, but they also willingly tell doctors about their most secret and intimate activities, habits, and relationships.

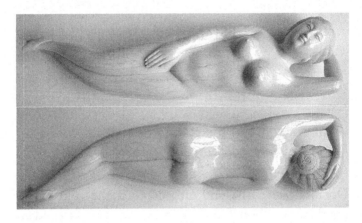

Given these circumstances, the doctor-patient relationship is such that doctors have a powerful role relative to their patients and are, in addition to being afforded a high level of respect, held to special behaviors and standards by convention, oath, and law. These standards include placing their patients' well-being and welfare above their personal or financial interests, prohibition of sexual relations between doctors and their patients, the treatment of patients with respect, and treating patients based on sound medical information and principles.

Despite the general good behavior and good intentions, patients can assume about doctors, patients should recognize that doctors are also human and might also be subject to modification of behavior depending upon the emotional content of their interaction with patients. It is clearly in the best interest of both patients and doctors to have positive doctor-patient interactions.

If a doctor perceives that the doctor-patient relationship is strained or hostile, or if a patient simply does not cooperate in following critical health advice, the doctor may formally end the relationship. This should involve the doctor discussing the situation with the patient and directing or referring the patient to another doctor for care. This should be documented in the patient's records, and the patient should receive a written notice to this effect. Failure to follow these guidelines, especially for a patient who requires ongoing care, could result in a doctor being accused of medical abandonment which is a breach of law.

In parallel to the above, should patients feel that their relationship with their doctor is strained, cold, or somehow not "normal" or "right," they definitely should consider changing their care to another doctor. Should patients not be able to change doctors, they must have a calm and frank discussion with their doctor about the doctor's "bedside manner" or the relationship as they see it. A poor relationship with your doctor can interfere with your response to therapy and might make you question your doctor's judgment and recommendations. Of course, implied in all of this is that as a patient, you take care to uphold your part in developing a good doctor-patient relationship. You probably do not want to be condescending, hostile, or sarcastic. Likewise, your doctor should not brush off or make light of your concerns, fail to explain things fully, or even seem to blame you for the problem. Do not think of yourself as a human-machine and of your doctor as a mechanic. Your body and mind and your doctor and therapies need to work together toward the aim of health.

CHAPTER 3

GENERALISTS AND SPECIALISTS

Five doctors went duck hunting one day. Included in the group were a general practitioner, a pediatrician, a psychiatrist, a surgeon, and a pathologist. After a time, a bird came winging overhead. The first to react was the general practitioner who raised his shotgun but then hesitated.

"I'm not quite sure it's a duck," he said. "I think that I will have to get a second opinion." And of course, by that time, the bird was long gone.

Another bird appeared in the sky soon thereafter. This time, the pediatrician drew a bead on it. He too, however, was unsure if it was really a duck in his sights, and besides, it might have babies. "I'll have to do some more investigations," he muttered, as the creature made good its escape.

Next to spy a bird flying was the sharp-eyed psychiatrist. Shotgun shouldered, he was more certain of his intended prey's identity. "Now, I know it's a duck, but does it know it's a duck?" The fortunate bird disappeared while the fellow wrestled with this dilemma.

Finally, a fourth fowl sped past, and this time the surgeon's weapon pointed skyward, and he fired without hesitation. BOOM! The surgeon lowered his smoking gun and turned nonchalantly to the pathologist beside him. "Go see if that was a duck, will you?"

https://public.websites.umich.edu/~bbowman/birds/humor/5docs.html accessed 2/9/24

What are the three fields in which primary care doctors are trained?

Which doctors do not treat patients?

Until the European Enlightenment (1685–1815), in the Western world, doctors were also charged with or were ascribed with what today might be called priestly duties. Illness, especially the specificity of "me being ill," was associated with a breach between the ill person and higher or godly power(s). Also, historically—for example, in the Egyptian and Roman imperial eras—doctors treated all manner of problems from injuries such as war wounds and burns to diseases such as infections and arthritis. However, in the European medieval period, the surgical approaches to medicine developed independently from the medical. Surgical doctors of that time developed from full-time barbers often living with or as monks, whose heads needed shaving. They also did bloodletting, cupping, amputations, and other surgeries. These so-called barber-surgeons were represented by the red and white (blood and bandages) striped poles still occasionally seen in association with barber shops.

Because of the introduction of anesthesia, surgery was able to develop and be taken fully into the sphere of doctors. Today, only in the most remote areas do physician generalists perform surgery beyond the most minor procedures.

Generalists who treated all manner of medical and surgical conditions, delivered babies, and treated children, were once known as "general doctors" or "family doctors" and might have had no training other than medical school. Generalists or primary care doctors are now considered to be those doctors whose training is in family medicine, internal medicine, or pediatrics. Broadly, medical doctors are divided into those who treat children (pediatricians), those who treat medical conditions specific to women (obstetricians and gynecologists), those who treat adults (internal medicine), and those who treat by surgery (surgeons). These are also the four main fields for clinical training of medical students. That is, medical students receive considerable training and exposure in pediatrics, obstetrics-gynecology, internal medicine, and surgery. The list of specialists and subspecialists is long and expanding with the growth in our knowledge and technological advances. Specialists include those in medical and surgical fields such as neurology and neurosurgery, and cardiology and cardiac surgery. The public does not know of all the specialists and subspecialists, and generalists act as sorters or triage officers treating the common problems and referring patients to the appropriate specialists as needed.

Another way doctors are organized is by those who do cosmetic medicine versus those do medical or noncosmetic medicine. Doctors who do solely cosmetic medicine, are mainly in the fields of dermatology and plastic surgery, doing procedures such as face lifts, hair transplants, treating wrinkles with nerve toxins and sagging faces with fillers, and revising scars, and removing tattoos. Cosmetic medicine is often referred to as "well" or "happy" medicine. While in most medical situations, patients want to return to "normal," in cosmetic situations, people aim to be "better than normal or ahead." Surgery aimed at repairing scars and other deformities is referred to as reconstructive or restorative surgery, is done mostly by plastic surgeons, and is only considered cosmetic in the broadest sense. Doctors, such as radiologists, pathologists, and anesthesiologists, have limited interaction with patients and participate in patient care by assisting or informing the treating doctor by way of providing anesthesia or laboratory and other diagnostic testing. Some doctors choose fields far removed from direct patient care, such as public health doctors, doctors who only do laboratory or preclinical research, doctors who work for drug companies, and doctors who become full-time medical directors or assume other major administrative roles.

Medical students and young medical school graduates choose to be generalists or specialists based on many personal factors, such as the influence of one of their professors, the perception of the lifestyle of the doctors in certain fields, or their enjoyment of the type of patients seen in a certain area (e.g., pediatricians deal with children). Generalists deal with a wide variety of patients and conditions and usually have more in-depth associations with patients, which is attractive to many students. Other students are attracted to the more limited but hands-on and quick-results nature of surgery, while others find the detective or diagnostic element of internal medicine especially appealing. Psychiatry offers a special population and a wide array of treatments including talk therapy, while the visual utilization of pattern recognition employed in pathology and radiology appeals to others.

Overall, when speaking of medical specialists, subspecialists, and even generalists, the implication is that the doctor has specific specialized training and that the doctor's training and skills are attested to or certified by boards such as the American Board of Internal Medicine or the American Board of Surgery. Specialty boards certify physicians based on their training having been in approved and certified by training centers and on written and sometimes oral examinations. Most boards now require recertification in about ten years. In the United States, there are twenty-four allopathic specialty boards representing forty specialties and eighty-eight subspecialties. Similarly, the osteopathic doctors certify twenty-seven primary specialties and forty-eight subspecialties. Most developed countries have similar ways of recognizing and certifying the training of specialists and subspecialists.

CHAPTER 4

CONSULTANTS, EXPERTS, SPECIALISTS, AND GENERALISTS

"An expert is somebody from out of town with slides"—Naomi Judd

"An expert is somebody who is more than Fifty miles from home, has no responsibility for implementing the advice he gives"—Edwin Meese

A physician, a civil engineer, and a consultant were arguing about what was the oldest profession in the world.

The physician remarked, "Well, in the Bible, it says that God created Eve from a rib taken out of Adam. This clearly required surgery, and so I can rightly claim that mine is the oldest profession in the world."

The civil engineer interrupted, and said, "But even earlier in the book of Genesis, it states that God created the order of the heavens and the earth from out of the chaos. This was the first and certainly the most spectacular application of civil engineering.

Therefore, fair doctor, you are wrong. Mine is the oldest profession in the world."

The consultant leaned back in her chair, smiled, and then said confidently, "Ah, but who do you think created the chaos?"

*https://www.glassdoor.com/Community/
consulting/63fbd88cacfb14004c180500 accessed 2/19/24*

What medical specialty cares for patients admitted to the hospital by their generalist?

What is the foremost advantage a consultant has over a generalist?

As recently as the 1950s, in the United States, there was a category of physicians known as general practitioners. They were also referred to as general doctors or family doctors but had less formal training for their roles than today's family practitioners. General practitioners were especially common in rural areas and were often either physicians who had begun practice after a single postgraduate year of internship or were general surgeons whose location precluded restricting their practices to surgery alone. General practitioners saw patients of all ages, and both sexes, made house calls, and knew their patients' families and much about their lives. The general doctor as the entry point to medical care has given way to more highly trained generalists: pediatricians (for children), obstetricians/gynecologists (for diseases of women), internists (internal medicine), and most recently family practitioners. These four, and in some health-care systems, nurse practitioners and physician assistants diagnose and treat most patients, at least initially. In health-care systems, these generalist doctors are often called gatekeepers since they control which patients are sent to specialists.

Specialist doctors care for a narrower spectrum of patients and diseases. Often they have training as generalists—for example, in pediatrics or internal medicine—and then have additional training to become subspecialists. For example, after several years of pediatrics training, some doctors might train in psychiatry and become pediatric psychiatrists. Another example would be someone who trained for several years to be an internist and then for another period of time to become a heart doctor (cardiologist); or training as a general surgeon and then becoming a transplantation surgeon. Other examples are emergency room doctors whose practice is limited to the emergency department and hospitalists, who care for people admitted to the hospital by their generalist.

While all doctors and specialist doctors are experts, some are more "expert" than others, and some of these doctors are primarily consultants. Experts and consultants have usually done and, often, are continuing to do research in their fields and, based on their publications and talks at scientific or medical meetings, have become recognized for their special knowledge and insights. Many experts and consultants work in medical schools where they can continue their investigative research, travel to conferences, and teach students in addition to consulting. Consultants are also often more experienced or senior physicians.

Currently, the phrase "second opinion" is often used when a patient seeks advice from a consultant or an expert. Second opinions are most often sought for cancers, especially rare cancers, and frequently involve not only clinical oncologists (doctors specializing in cancer treatment) but also radiologists and pathologists. Second opinions are also sought or sometimes required before deciding to proceed with certain surgeries. Consultants of all types are considered to be independent of the doctor with primary responsibility for the patient.

Consultants have certain, not often recognized, advantages in diagnosing and treating or recommending treatments to patients. Foremost among these advantages is that patients referred to them have already been found to not have the common explanations or diagnoses for their situation. Also, the patients will most likely be suffering a condition in the specialist's sphere of expertise. Importantly, the consultant will have a team of people, both clinicians and scientists, to assist in making a diagnosis and developing or even administering treatments. In addition, consultants often have special resources and technologies that are sometimes in the developmental stage or are not widely available. Having been in the consulting position for some time, consultants will also have seen, diagnosed, and treated patients with many of the rare conditions or circumstances that occur in their specialty. Consultants are also alert to being sent patients who are in actuality, now suffering mostly, or even entirely, the side effects produced by treatments given for their initial condition.

Consultants, experts, and specialists are naturally at risk of seeing all problems through their specialty lenses. While this is usually good, it can on occasion produce the wrong result. Such is captured in the phrase, when you go to a meat market, you're going to get meat.

Finally, it should be noted, that many of the doctors who are consultants for individual patients, are also consultants to related fields such as pharmaceutical and medical device companies, especially in assisting with new drug or medical device development or new uses for already marketed products . Often, the consultants have done the groundwork that has led to work on developing a new drug or new use. Physicians also are consultants to important government agencies such as the Food and Drug Administration and the National Institutes of Health. Physician consultants also assist companies to teach doctors and nurses about new drugs and devices and in this capacity may be known as Key Opinion Leaders or KOLs. These activities allow consultants to be abreast of new options and ideas in their fields, which may also be helpful for their patients.

CHAPTER 5

SURGEONS (SURGEON DOCTORS)

What is the difference between God and a surgeon? God doesn't think he's a surgeon.

http://folklore.usc.edu/the-difference-between-god-and-a-surgeon/ accessed 2/21/24

Which national regulatory body assures that new surgical procedures are better than sham or placebo surgeries?

As noted earlier, the surgical approach to disease, at least in the European world, grew from barbers who started doing bloodletting and other minor procedures. With the discovery of anesthesia, surgery was able to join and augment the more scholarly, although often wrong, medical approaches of doctors.

Today surgeons are medical school graduates (physicians) who have additional special training, usually several years, in doing surgery. They may be generalists (general surgeons) who do a broad range of common surgeries such as appendectomies, or they are surgical subspecialists such as neurosurgeons. Surgical subspecialists have had additional training beyond general surgery and limit their surgeries to a given organ or type of surgery—for example, vascular surgery. While surgeons also treat patients with medications, their skill at removing and repairing tissues by physical means is what separates them from other doctors. Surgeons work in tandem with anesthesiologists who keep patients unconscious and pain-free during the surgical procedure. Surgeons also depend on surgical or operating nurses and other support services. Surgery is inherently somewhat dramatic, often producing profound effects quickly. This contrasts with the most often slower and less dramatic results produced by taking medications or nonsurgical-physical and manipulative therapies. Training in surgery is perhaps the most rigorous and demanding of all specialties and requires teamwork, coordination and cooperation far beyond the ordinary.

The personality that leads to a doctor preferring a field where often dramatic results are produced quickly by dexterous hands on patients who are unconscious is part of what leads to the characterizations of surgeons as people who are humorously suggested to be too confident, too aggressive, too impatient, and too certain that surgery is the answer. While such tongue in cheek characterizations were never universally true, surgeons of today are trained in less severe circumstances and are even less likely to fit the stereotypic mold of the past. Personality aside, surgeons produce remarkable, dramatic, lifesaving and life changing procedures. Among the many examples are minimally invasive laparoscopic and robotic-assisted surgeries and organ transplant.

Although unrelated to surgeons per se, another feature separating the surgical field from the medical field is that there is no national regulatory body assuring that surgical treatments are better and safer than placebo (sham) or nonsurgical treatments or the standard of the moment. By contrast, before drugs (and devices) are allowed to be sold on the US market, they must be approved as safe and effective by the Food and Drug Administration (FDA). The importance of such approval is illustrated by the famous study of the once widespread use of a surgical procedure known as "internal mammary artery ligation" for the treatment of angina (pain from blocked blood flow to the heart). In this procedure, the patient's chest was opened and vessels tied off to force more blood through the patient's coronary arteries and heart. Although not required by law, when studies were finally done comparing internal mammary artery ligation to sham surgery (opening the patient's chest but not tying of the blood vessels) the therapeutic results were the same! (*N Engl J* Med. 1959;260(22):1115-1118). Similar results have been found with sham, control treatments for other surgical therapies such as osteoarthritis of the knees. (N *Engl J Med.* 2002;347(2):81-88).

FDA approval is necessary to sell new, complex medical devices, and when new devices are needed for a new operation—the FDA essentially ensures the safety and efficacy of the new surgical approach by approving the device.

CHAPTER 6

DOCTORS AND THERAPY

Some years ago in London, an elderly woman told her doctor that she was invited to go on safari in East Africa, in an area several hundred miles from the nearest doctor. She wanted to know if he felt it was safe for her to accept. The doctor told her that while the difference between being treated by a good doctor and a bad doctor was enormous, the difference between having no doctor and a good doctor could hardly be measured. —*Sir William Osler*

(Author's note: For much of recorded history, this might well have been the case.)

In one study, participants were split into three groups. The first group was told they would receive a treatment for erectile dysfunction, the second group was told they would receive either a placebo or an actual treatment, and the third group was told they would receive a placebo.

All three groups were, in fact, given placebo starch tablets, but the erectile dysfunction in all three groups improved significantly without any differences between the three groups.

J Sex Med. 2009 Dec;6(12):3440-8.

Placebo responses have also been linked to increases in dopamine and opioid receptor activity. Both of these chemicals are involved in reward and motivation pathways in the brain. Conversely, nocebos have been found to reduce dopamine and opioid receptor activity.

https://www.medicalnewstoday.com/articles/306437#what-is-the-placebo-effect Accessed 2/21/24

Do placebos work when patients know it is a placebo?

How often are doctors' diagnoses estimated to be wrong/right?

It is best to begin understanding doctors' approaches to therapy by understanding placebos and the placebo effect. The placebo popularly known as a "sugar pill" produces effects that can be ascribed to the act of taking the pill, not to the chemical action of the pill's contents. Placebos are not only sugar pills. For example, as mentioned earlier, sham surgery where an incision is made and sutured closed is a placebo, as is the application of a cream without the active or test agent. The word placebo derives from the Latin verb placeo, which means "I will please," which is the aim of the placebo. Placebo effects are produced by our minds, and there is evidence suggesting that in response to the sugar pill or other placebo stimulus, such as sham therapy, our brains release chemicals that produce the so-called placebo effect.

Placebos have been and are used extensively in tests to prove that a drug or a device or some other intervention is effective. In fact, US law basically defines a drug or intervention as effective if it produces the desired effect more often or better than a placebo. Depending upon the disease, placebo responses will be in the 20 to 40 percent range. There is clear experimental evidence that placebos work even when the recipient is told that "this is a sugar or placebo pill." Placebos given with the subject's understanding that they are being given placebos are known as "open placebos."

The reason it is important to understand that placebos, including for example mock surgery for arthritic knees or coronary heart disease, work is that doctors themselves and medical interventions have a clinically significant degree of effectiveness based solely on the placebo effect. Thus patients, in fact, do improve simply by making an appointment to see the doctor. Doctors are and have always been extremely good at producing placebo effects. It is not only the doctor as a person but the entire setting. The recognition that this is a place for treating and healing, the office or hospital, the front desk and nurse, the waiting room, the respect for the physician and the formal suit of the past, the white coat or scrub suit of the present, all cooperate to induce a healing or favorable response. This effect is quite independent of the pharmacological effect of a medication or the physical effect of surgery.

Understanding the therapeutic power of physicians and the entire medical environment helps one understand the importance of choosing doctors with the personality or approach in which you have confidence and environments that build confidence in you or those to be treated. Although doctors are quite familiar with the placebo effect of pills and injections, they often fail to recognize the degree to which they personally and their environments are placebos.

As noted, to be recognized as a drug (an active agent) by the FDA, the agent must be better able to produce a desired therapeutic effect than a placebo. To prove such to the FDA, candidate drugs are tested in people who have the condition the drug is intended to treat, and the effect is compared to the effect produced by a placebo in people who have the same condition. In a surprising percentage of cases, the candidate or would-be drug fails to be better. In fact, the power of placebos is such that they also can cause side effects, especially if side effects are expected or suggested. For example, subjects who were told that the test agent could cause gastrointestinal effects such as nausea were six times more likely to withdraw from studies with GI effects. This negative effect of a sugar pill is called the "nocebo" effect.

Perhaps, the most famous dictum in medicine is "first, do no harm." It is also rendered as "above all do no harm." It is a principle that is universally taught to all students in the health-care field and is found in the Hippocratic oath as a pledge to "abstain from doing harm." This concern is large in doctors' assessments of any treatment or intervention recommendations they make. Such concern for safety is often a source of frustration for patients in their quest for solutions.

Medications, surgeries, and other treatment technologies have become more powerful over the last eighty years. Medicines especially have offered a degree of biological activity unknown before 1900. Unfortunately, their bioactivities are not specific enough to induce only the desired effects but rather may also produce undesired or so-called side effects. Part of the doctor's skill comes in the ability to "fit" these agents or contemporary surgeries, radiation therapies, and other physical treatments to the patient's circumstances so as to obtain the maximum therapeutic effect with the least potential for side effects. Drugs and other technologies are approved to sell and use in the medical field based on what is called the benefit-to-risk ratio. That is, the FDA not only requires proof of therapeutic activity greater than a placebo but also requires the benefits of a drug or technology to outweigh the potential risks to patients. Obviously, greater risk can be taken in treating dire or life-threatening conditions. Put another way, when the benefit such as avoiding death is great, FDA approval may be granted even though the treatment has the potential to cause serious side effects. This benefit-to-risk ratio or trade-off also guides physicians in their approach to treating patients. Your doctor will initially recommend treatments that are the most safe. At one extreme, when the condition is known to end or clear up without treatment (self-limited), only the safest, symptomatic treatment will be suggested. At the other end of the spectrum, when the condition or situation is life-threatening, treatments that may have serious adverse or side effects may be prescribed. Obviously, when the safest treatments fail, and the condition does not improve or resolve on its own, doctors move on to prescribe medicines or treatments that are more difficult (i.e., may demand more visits or courses), have greater potential for side effects, and may even require tests to monitor for side effects.

Generally, doctors will not offer treatments that are likely to be harmful. However, as knowledge is acquired, a treatment once thought to have benefits that warranted the risk of side or harmful effects may be found to, in fact, do more harm than good or be only harmful. An example from the past is the therapy known as bleeding or bloodletting. This practice of the physician or barber in which veins in the upper limb are cut to release blood was thought to restore the balance of the body's humors, blood being one of the four humors. Subsequently, bloodletting was thought to be helpful for inflammatory diseases where tissue redness and/or warmth was thought to indicate too much blood—hence the treatment to let or reduce the amount of blood by bleeding. We now understand that bleeding, with a rare exception for people with too much iron, is not helpful and in most situations probably harmful.

Overall, the treatments doctors prescribe will depend on the diagnosis or nature of the patient's condition. When doctors cannot determine a specific diagnosis or cause, they often simply prescribe medicines or treatments that combat or treat the symptoms. Between the body's innate healing capacity, the placebo effect, and various drug and surgical treatments, doctors are very often successful. The fact that most doctors treat the most common conditions in their fields most of the time means they become very good at it. However, doctors can and do make mistakes.

The physician can bury his mistakes, but the architect can only advise his client to plant vines. —Frank Lloyd Wright

The "mistakes" of doctors are usually divided into two categories: medical mistakes and thinking errors. The best-known and the most common of the thinking errors is the category known as diagnostic errors. Medical mistakes are matters such as removing the wrong organ (wrong side surgery) or prescribing the wrong dose of a medicine.

Diagnostic errors are matters of failure to properly put together a patient's signs and symptoms (misdiagnosis or delayed diagnosis) and are often the result of biased thinking. Biased thinking or so-called cognitive biases are unconscious. Biases affect a doctor's thinking, hence diagnoses, and therefore therapies. The most common biases affecting doctor's thinking are anchoring bias— the tendency to diagnose a condition in a new patient that fits with the doctor's most common or recent experience; confirmation bias—the tendency to accept and find proof of whatever diagnosis the doctor instantly believes best or was sent in the referral information; and availability bias—believing the treatment most available to the doctor is the best treatment (e.g., the doctor has expertise with a certain laser).

Overall doctors are usually accurate in their diagnoses, but it is estimated that about 10 percent of their diagnoses are wrong. When a doctor cannot make a diagnosis or the patient has not improved despite the treatments, a referral is commonly made, usually to a consultant, someone with greater expertise in the area the doctor believes the answer or diagnosis lies. The doctor to whom the patient is sent is known as the consultant because the referring doctor is asking for or consulting on the situation or the "case." Often, the consultant will advise the referring physician who will resume care of the patient but will consider or follow the wisdom and advice of the consultant. Alternately, the consultant may become the patient's physician because of having the latest or best treatment technology or experience with the latest drug or drug combination. Of course, many times patients take the initiative of seeking alternative care by making their own appointment to see another physician or asking their primary or current doctor for a referral. Doctors should be quite open to requests from patients for a referral. Should they not be open to referring a patient when asked, patients and their families should definitely be suspicious and should seek another opinion on their own.

Finally, a word of caution about rushing to procedures or treatments that have the potential for harm. Perhaps this message is best conveyed in the phrase, "Don't just do something, stand there." Time is often on the side of healing, and medications often need to be adjusted rather than abandoned. Even when a treatment is abandoned, another medication, even of the same class, may work for some patients while not for other patients. That is, medications often need to be tried and fitted to each patient. Also, patients need to realize that medications not taken or not taken as prescribed will not work, at least pharmacologically.

CHAPTER 7

DOCTORS, DECISIONS, AND DATA

What is meant by "evidence-based medicine?"

What do doctors do if they do not have direct evidence to answer a patient's questions?

Doctors make diagnoses, and decisions, give advice, or respond to patients' questions with suggestions hundreds of times a day. For most doctors, the primary diagnoses they make will be from among about the ten most common diagnoses in their field. Once the patient's diagnosis or problem is clearly not among the most common for that physician or not one the physician can easily deal with, a referral is suggested or made. For returning or follow-up patients, diagnoses and decisions will relate to the response to therapy such as side effects, lack of sufficient response, and so forth. Regarding the many questions that doctors are asked, often there is no study or explicit information on the specific question or issue for the patient and his or her circumstances. For example, if a cardiologist is asked if a fifty-three-year-old woman patient with a recent heart attack should abstain from visiting her grandchildren at her son and daughter-in-law's house because all entrances to the house require climbing two flights of stairs, the answer will be based on related information but not a study of this specific situation. People who become doctors are comfortable with this role of translating science-based information or new technologies to the specific circumstances of their patients. People who select other fields, especially those that are science-based, might not be comfortable giving so much advice based on so little clear evidence. In general, a doctor's advice and answers are based on what they have been taught, their experience (empiric information), and scientifically derived information bearing directly or indirectly on the decision or question.

The phrase "evidence-based medicine" now reflects the desire to base medical decisions and advice upon information derived from controlled human studies. To some extent, it is a prejudicial phrase because it presupposes doctors might not base their decisions on data. However, a more generous, and I believe more accurate view, is that this phrase is intended to emphasize the need to make primary the results of human studies bearing on the decisions and advice doctors make and give.

Regarding evidence or data, doctors are the recipients of a constant cascade of information. New findings are reported by email, print, lectures, and videos. Both basic science and clinical (human) research results compete for the doctor's attention. New information comes to doctors from general and specialty journals, medical meetings, local and national societies, hospitals, medical boards, licensing bodies, and other government sources. And of course, patients bring information to their doctors which should be welcomed by the doctors as a point of discussion as well as education. The half-life of new medical knowledge is now estimated to be about two years. Clearly, patients want their doctors to be alert to and able to use new findings to their benefit. However, more than a few observers have commented that their doctors might be dangerous after learning a few new things at a medical meeting! There is an age-old tension between the desire to be cared for by a young doctor perceived to be most up-to-date and an older doctor considered to be tempered by experience. At least regarding the basic underlying knowledge, AI might soon provide a leveling effect.

However, current hopes for the role of artificial intelligence (AI) in medical diagnosis and decision-making might suggest to some observers and commentators that computers and AI might displace or supplant doctors in diagnosing and advising on therapy and behavior. However, the doctor's role is not only to make the proper diagnosis but also to explain to patients and relate treatment(s) and behavioral advice to the individual patient. It is unlikely that AI will be able to do this on a case-by-case basis. The role of translating new technological medical information to the specificity and circumstances of each patient will undoubtedly endure, as it has done historically. Importantly, the human interaction and the so-called "laying on of hands," or touching and examining has a soothing and therapeutic effect and offers many diagnostic clues and cues regarding a patient's reaction to the idea of different therapies. All of this is unlikely to be afforded by interaction with technology. For example, artificial intelligence is unlikely to compete in the "laying on of hands" arena. AI is, however, likely to relieve doctors of the current need to physically document their patient interactions and allow more effective visits with a more personal doctor-patient interaction in addition to being a valuable aide in making diagnoses and finding therapies.

CHAPTER 8

COSMETIC SURGERY AND COSMETIC MEDICINE

Looking fifty is great if you're sixty.
—Joan Rivers

How do you hide a $100 bill from a surgeon?
Put it in a textbook.
How do you hide $100 from an internist?
Put it under the patient's gown.
How do you hide $100 from a radiologist?
Give it to the patient.
How do you hide it from a plastic surgeon?
You can't
—Unknown

Which specialists practice cosmetic medicine?

What is another name for restorative surgery?

What is body dysmorphic disorder?

Cosmetic surgery and cosmetic medicine are practiced by doctors from many specialties. In the popular mind, plastic surgeons rank foremost, and as indicated in the epigram, the economic basis for their activities is often the source of popular humor.

One of the reasons different specialties are involved in cosmetic medicine is that "cosmetic" refers both to improving the normal appearance and to restoring abnormal appearances. Birth defects—for example, cleft lips and hemangiomas—burn scars and contractions, and severe war or traumatic injuries are among the problems corrected or improved by restorative or reconstructive surgery. Breast implantation following breast cancer surgery is another example of restorative surgery. By contrast, surgical procedures aimed at improving appearance include surgeries such as face and buttock lifts, hair transplantation, and nose surgery (rhinoplasty). Injections of botulinum toxin (e.g. Botox) and wrinkle fillers as well as laser resurfacing and hair and tattoo removal are among the so-called nonsurgical cosmetic procedures. Plastic surgeons are best known for doing both reconstructive and cosmetic surgery/medicine. The very name "plastic surgery" suggests elegance in outcome as compared to most specialty names, which focus on the tissue or organ. In addition to plastic surgeons, dermatologists, dental surgeons, nose and throat doctors, and obstetric and gynecologic doctors also do cosmetic surgery and procedures, especially botulinum toxin injections.

Cosmetic medicine is often called "happy medicine" because the results are aimed at "getting you ahead" rather than the usual goal of "just" being well or normal again. However, in the United States, doctors who do cosmetic medicine and surgery are considered at high risk for lawsuits and pay especially high prices for insurance. Doctors who do cosmetic medicine must also be able to assess and adjust patient expectations to what is possible rather than what is hoped for or expected based on popular literature. In addition, doctors doing cosmetic medicine must be alert to patients who are pathologically focused on their appearance, the so-called "body dysmorphic disorder."

CHAPTER 9

PUBLIC HEALTH DOCTORS AND PUBLIC HEALTH

What are some of the fields of knowledge that public health doctors study?

For whom do public health doctors usually work?

Whereas most doctors deal with patients one at a time, public health doctors deal with populations rather than with individuals. Not all public health professionals are physicians. Some have PhDs or master's degrees in public health. Physicians who specialize in public health are trained in the same manner as other doctors but ultimately take additional training or learn on the job to become public health specialists. Public health doctors have special expertise in fields such as epidemiology, environmental health, biostatistics, behavioral science, and health services administration. During the recent COVID-19 pandemic, both national and local public health officials, most of whom were doctors, became known to the public by way of the various restrictions and closures they imposed.

While some public health doctors do treat individual patients in their role as public health doctors, they are concerned with matters such as epidemics of infectious or other diseases, air and water quality, food quality, and endemic diseases such as tuberculosis and sexually transmitted diseases. Public health doctors usually work for a government agency at levels ranging from cities to counties, states, and national governments—for example, the US Centers for Disease Control and international organizations such as the World Health Organization.

CHAPTER 10

DOCTOR'S DRESS

Why are doctors' scrub suits and surgical drapes green or blue?

In the Middle Ages, doctors wore black gowns and hoods. Depending on the circumstances, they might have also worn long beaklike masks containing dried plants with pleasant smells in order to let them deal with foul-smelling conditions. Since at that time, it was thought that some diseases, such as plague, might be caused by bad air, doctors also hoped that the masks would protect them. These masks were reminiscent of ducks' beaks (see Fig) and are thought by some people to be the basis for the disparaging term "quacks" being applied to some doctors. Doctors subsequently started wearing more formal streetwear but protected their clothing with aprons when doing surgery. Before the recognition of bacteria, doctors would often wear the same clothing while moving from doing autopsies to delivering babies in the hospital. The fact that wealthy women whose babies were delivered in the hospital had more infections and deaths compared to poor women who delivered at home was one of the clues leading to an understanding of infection and its transmission. By the 1940s, doctors had started wearing white coats over their formal suits, at least in the hospital. Today, physicians often wear white coats over semiformal clothing or scrubs or scrubs alone. Scrubs were originally developed to wear during surgery. They were deliberately made either green or blue in order to avoid visual insensitivity to various red colors that might occur when looking at a bloody surgical field. Surgical gowns are also made of the same colors for this reason.

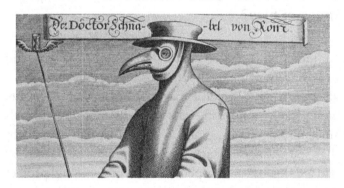

How doctors dress is quite important to patients even if this importance is subliminal. Large surveys of patients have shown greater satisfaction with doctors who dress more formally. Dress and environment play important roles in the placebo effect that doctors have. Pediatricians often avoid wearing ties or they wear bowties since infants may pee or vomit on them, and children often grab hold of long neckties with dirty hands!

CHAPTER 11

DOCTORS, EXTRA SMART PATIENTS, RELATIVES AND FRIENDS, AND CONCIERGE MEDICINE

"Great intelligence, and high position in a patient, bear no relation to his understanding of medical problems." ~Dr. Mark M. Ravitch

Is it illegal for doctors to refuse to give patients the treatments they ask for?

What are the advantages of retainer medicine?

Very intelligent and/or prominent patients are most often a joy, especially pleasant, and interesting for doctors. Because of the key and unusual roles these patients often play, they offer interesting conversations, and many have already researched their medical situation. But despite their success in other fields, and even having accumulated a good deal of information on their own, they are not able to judge the relative importance of what they have learned. A few patients in this category operate on the proposition that since they are very bright and have assumed leadership positions based partly on their mental capacity, they should also be in charge of their care. They are likely to have researched what they presume is their problem and are often insistent on treatments they have recently read about.

Doctors, by convention and law, are accountable for making proper diagnoses and offering the best and safest treatments for the patient's circumstances. As such, doctors cannot simply act as conduits or implementors of the patient's conclusions and desires of the moment. This dynamic is quite different from the so-called "buyer-beware" set of circumstances operative in many purchases. That is, convention, ethics, and the law recognize that even the brightest lay people are untrained in understanding medical circumstances and medical literature. Not only are they unlikely to be able to fully comprehend the biomedical circumstances, but their judgments and conclusions are colored and biased by their emotional reaction to their circumstances. This impairment of objectivity and judgment occurs to all patients, and even to doctors themselves as testified to by observations such as, "The doctor who treats himself has a fool for a patient," from Sir William Osler, a famous physician educator. Because of emotional involvement in thinking and judgment, doctors are ethically constrained from treating immediate family members, relatives, and even close friends. As noted elsewhere, doctoring is largely practiced patient by patient and not easily scaled up. Patients and circumstances are all unique.

Extra-bright and prominent patients who are most likely to come to the doctor-patient relationship with a sense of being in charge of their care may be viewed by doctors as somewhat burdensome, especially given the time constraints of medical practices within large corporate health-care organizations. In the corporatized systems, patients who are accepting of a benign paternalism most "fit" into the circumstances of the system. Dissatisfaction with the short time that the doctors are "allowed" to spend with patients has led some doctors to a type of practice known as concierge medicine. In this type of practice, primary care doctors agree to provide care to only a limited number of patients who pay an annual fee, which is independent of health insurance that may or may not be used in the concierge setup. This limited-load type practice lets the doctor know the patients very well, provide same-day appointments, spend generous amounts of time at each visit, be readily available by phone and text, do preventive care, and so forth. This relationship is also called retainer medicine.

CHAPTER **12**

DOCTOR-PATIENT RELATIONSHIP

What are some legal reasons doctors can stop caring for a patient?

What are the requirements to sue for malpractice?

The doctor-patient relationship is a legally formal relationship or contract, although doctors and patients usually don't think of it that way. The actual legalities or terms of the "contract" may vary with the circumstances and place, but at its core, doctors are responsible for providing proper care, maintaining confidentiality, and respecting and not abandoning patients. Patients understand that they have accepted the doctor as their doctor and are directly or indirectly responsible for the financials of the contract. However, such a contractual definition fails to describe the intense and deep nature of the doctor-patient relationship. Patients often reveal secrets, worries, and fears to physicians that they have not yet disclosed to friends or family members. Placing trust in a doctor helps them maintain or regain their health and well-being.

Both the doctor and the patient may break their contract. For patients, it simply requires going to another physician. Doctors require specific reasons and must notify the patients in writing and offer them an alternative caregiver. Reasons allowed for doctors to break the contract include doctors retiring or moving, patients not paying bills, patients being rude or obnoxious, patients not keeping appointments, and patients not following recommendations. Doctors cannot break the contract for reasons of race, color, national origin, sexual orientation, and so forth.

Doctors are aware that they are subject to lawsuits brought by patients. These lawsuits are broadly called malpractice lawsuits. While rare in the past, malpractice lawsuits are now relatively common depending a great deal upon medical specialty. In some specialties (e.g. orthopedic surgery, ob-gyn, and plastic surgery), over 70 percent of the doctors have been sued. Malpractice lawsuits require proof of four major elements: there must be a doctor-patient relationship, the doctor must have failed to offer care at the community level, the failure must have caused injury, and the injury has resulted in damages that have financial consequences. Laws exempt doctors from lawsuits when they are acting as good Samaritans—for example, caring for people on the site immediately after an automobile accident. Doctors usually know which sets of circumstances in their field are most at risk for or likely to produce a malpractice lawsuit. Doctors also realize that they or their employers pay a great deal for malpractice insurance. Nevertheless, most doctors are emotionally unprepared for being sued for malpractice. They think of themselves as the good guys and have been considered to be and treated as such throughout their careers. Being charged as a bad guy or someone who did not meet the standard is hard for them to process or accept. Most have considerable anxiety and many need treatment for anxiety or depression during the long process of dealing with and resolving a malpractice suit.

CHAPTER 13

WHO BECOME DOCTORS

A college physics professor was explaining a particularly complicated concept to his class when a pre-med student interrupted him. "Why do we have to learn this stuff?" the frustrated student blurted out. "To save lives," the professor responded, before continuing the lecture. A few minutes later, the student spoke up again. "So how does physics save lives?" The professor stared at the student without saying a word. "Physics saves lives," he finally continued, "because it keeps the idiots out of medical school."

https://www.reddit.com/r/Jokes/comments/uoptvs/life_saving/ accessed 2/21/24.

What is the average debt of graduating U.S. medical students?

Are most doctors employees or self-employed?

In the US, becoming a doctor requires high academic skills and is quite expensive. After receiving a bachelor's degree, which usually takes about four years, medical students study four more years. The first two years are mostly classroom learning. The last two years are spent learning by doing and observing in clinics and in-patient settings under the supervision of clinical faculty doctors, most often in health centers known as "teaching hospitals."

These medical-school-affiliated teaching institutions are usually sites of tertiary or final level health care and attract the most extreme or severe health situations. As such, they afford an excellent setting for training doctors and other health-care professionals who learn about diseases by seeing them in their extreme form. About 40 percent of students who apply are admitted to medical school. The average debt of graduating medical students is about $200,000. Following medical school, graduates spend one to six additional years doing clinical training in general or specialty training. Therefore, people who become doctors will be bright, disciplined, and hard workers who are studious, able to defer gratification, and whose next stage in life has been clear and creates little anxiety. They are usually from the middle and less disadvantaged elements of society, and because of the time devoted to study and work, they have often been out of the mainstream of life as known to others in their age group. They have not faced rejection or some of the ordinary experiences of many young people "getting started." They will also be confident, having had tremendous academic success. And perhaps, in some measure because of their success in the academic arena, those who become doctors are very much able to make decisions. Although often somewhat protected and privileged, medical students are quickly exposed to the physical and behavioral reality of the human condition. Gory sights and smells and irrational and psychotic behavior are seen and dealt with early in training. Both by formal training and by experience "in the trenches," doctors are able to separate their emotional response to disease and sick people from the needed analytic determination of causes and best treatments. While important, to some extent this emotional distancing may result in a less empathetic approach than might be desired by some patients and families in some circumstances. To the extent that empathy depends on being able to personally identify with a patient's situation, the somewhat homogeneously middle-class background of most doctors might limit their empathy.

People who become doctors like and are good at understanding science. They are also high-energy people who can concentrate on their studies and are able to defer many of the good times of youth and money-making in favor of study and training. They are attracted to the idea of helping people and "doing well by doing good." Historically, doctors did not work for or in large organizations and were often their own bosses. In the recent past, that opportunity was also an attraction.

However, today most doctors work in groups and often in large organizations, and while they are still key players, they are not truly independent operators. This has proven to be an attraction to many who do not wish to be involved with the administration or the finances required of the solo or small practice situations and who prefer to have more time-off opportunities—for example, for maternity leave. That is to say, people who become doctors today are comfortable with being employees, and having less demanding and more predictable schedules than their predecessors.

As mentioned earlier, doctors are comfortable making hundreds of decisions daily, often with thin evidence or only extrapolations from experiential nonclinical evidence for their recommendations. Science-liking students who prefer more precision often gravitate toward becoming PhD researchers rather than physicians. Those choosing to become physicians are generally natural people connectors and people touchers. This is also the case for nurses and others involved in health care. However, people who identify too strongly with the emotions of others and are adversely affected by others' problems and sufferings will not be comfortable as physicians. Some medical students do initially suffer from their emotional response to their patient's circumstances and suffering, and many medical students go through a period of thinking that they are suffering from one of the diseases they are studying. On occasions, such students decide not to become doctors. However, most students adjust and develop a clear idea of who has the disease. This is important since it allows a certain required objectivity when making diagnoses and recommending the next steps. Generally, doctors will know what to do in each patient's circumstances and disease stage.

CHAPTER 14

PHYSICIAN ASSISTANTS

What are two common types of nurse specialists?

Are physician assistants allowed to do surgery on patients?

Physicians are assisted by many people who, for example, make appointments, deal with billing, and by people who do technical procedures such as X-rays and sonograms, and people who do physical and occupational therapy. However, it is mostly nurses who assist with direct medical care in hospital and outpatient settings. There are many types and levels of nurses indicating different degrees and types of training. Those with the least training are certified nursing assistants (CNA) and licensed practical nurses (LPN). They usually work in hospitals and nursing homes under the supervision of registered nurses (RN). Advanced practice nurses (APN) and doctors of nursing practice (DNP) are more advanced and, depending on the state and local circumstances, practice independently or almost independently. Nurses, especially APNs, often have special areas or specialties, such as nurse midwives and nurse anesthetists. Nurse practitioners are also APNs but have training specific to their being able to diagnose and treat patients independently. Their degree of independence and range of activities will vary depending on state law.

Physician assistants, also known as physician associates, are a specific category of assistants who have special training and are licensed by the state. They do not have training or a background in nursing, and many must "practice" with the supervision or availability of a licensed physician either in the same building or contactable by phone. Physician assistants(PA) are allowed to assist in very specific ways defined somewhat differently in each state. For example, in California, PAs take histories, do physical examinations, order tests, make diagnoses, give injections, do minor surgery, and order medications as authorized by a doctor.

In the military, doctors are also assisted by medics (army and air force) or corpsmen (navy). While they most often work under the supervision of doctors, they may be semiautonomous depending upon the circumstances, especially on the battlefield.

The wide array of a doctor's assistants, including nurse practitioners and physician associates, is a somewhat recent advent. The long history of satisfaction with care provided by medics and corpsmen to those serving in the military and military families, coupled with the increased ability of medical care to be effective and the inherent relative doctor shortage, has led to a general openness and acceptance of care given by these physician assistants. Generally, the assistants who offer care more or less independently are primarily charged with caring for patients with routine or clear-cut conditions or circumstances. Part of their skill is to recognize when a patient's problems are beyond their ability. In systems where there is a physician shortage, APNs and PAs are often the primary caregivers and functionally control to which doctor(s) patients are then referred. Highly trained APNs and PAs being the de facto doctors or primary caregivers is likely to be more common in the future. In such circumstances, patients should take the same care to be comfortable and have confidence in their non-physician caregiver as is recommended for selecting their doctor.

Regarding the care given by nurses and other physician assistants, the legal burden for proper diagnosis and care rests largely with doctors and on occasion with hospitals. Certainly, in some instances, patients can be confused about who is responsible for their care. In extreme situations, responsibility is ultimately determined by way of legal proceedings.

CHAPTER 15

THE MEDICAL ENVIRONMENT
IN THE UNITED STATES

As a Canadian, every time I hear a bad joke
about being Canadian, I go right to the hospital
and get my feelings checked for free.
https://www.eatliver.com/canada/ accessed 2/21/24

Overheard this at the hospital:
Phlebotomist: "I'm here to draw some blood."
Patient: "But I just received blood yesterday."
Phlebotomist: "You didn't think you'd get to keep it, did you?"

https://forum.diabetes.org.uk/boards/threads/terrible-
terrible-jokes.109443/page-8 accessed 2/23/24

What percentage of health expenditures in the United States is for drugs?

What percentage of the health care budget is spent to pay doctors?

What percentage of drugs are generic?

Overall, today doctors practice in an environment that allows them tremendous opportunity to help their patients and the public. The "system," however, has a high degree of bureaucratization and costs which are too great for some portions of the population.

The medical or health-care world is very large. Nearly 20 percent, one of every five dollars, of all spending in the United States is on health or health care (in 1970 it was 6 percent). In other rich countries, the percentage of national spending is close to or slightly above 10 percent. Higher payments to hospitals and doctors, higher drug costs, administrative and insurance costs, and the cost of defensive medicine, tests, and treatments aimed at avoiding lawsuits, are among the reasons for this cost disparity. While doctors are the key players in determining what care is needed for patients, and hence how the money will be spent, they are not themselves the most expensive part of the system. Most of the costs, 35 percent, come from hospital expenses, while doctors account for 20 percent and drugs for 10 percent of health-care expenditures. The federal government pays for about 30 percent of all medical expenses, individuals pay about 30 percent, private insurance pays about 20 percent, and state and local governments pay about 15 percent.

As of September 2021, there were just over one million practicing physicians in the United States. This is about three doctors per one thousand people. About 90 percent of doctors live and work in urban or suburban areas where about 80 percent of the population lives. For some time, the number of women becoming doctors has been increasing, and at present the number of women in medical school is slightly greater than the number of men. However, there are still more male than female doctors, about 1.8 to 1.0.

Medical education in the United States is very expensive. Most medical students graduate with over $200,000 in debt. Doctors are, however, very well paid, having on average the highest-paid job in the US. Nevertheless, a doctor's pay or income will vary considerably depending upon the type of medicine or specialty the doctor practices and the place or system in which they practice. Certain specialties, such as family medicine, internal medicine, and pediatrics are poorly paid relative to others' specialties, such as ophthalmology, orthopedic surgery, and anesthesiology. Doctors may work as totally independent practitioners, in so-called private practices, or as employees. Private practices (most often fee-for-service practices) may have only one doctor, or a solo practitioner, or they may have many doctors either all in the same field or in different fields. Some of these doctors may be owners of the practice while others are employees, usually expecting to become owners over time.

At the other end of the spectrum, doctors may be full-time employees such as those employed by universities or health-care systems such as Kaiser Health, the armed forces, or the Veterans Administration hospital system. In general, doctors who want to avoid the administrative components of practicing medicine, such as billing and collecting, patient appointments, and administration of employees, will prefer to work for large health-care systems, including health maintenance organizations. Working in these systems also mitigates the problem of being on call for patients during off-hours. Generally, full-time employee doctors will have somewhat lower incomes than the incomes of doctors in the so-called private sector. However, this difference is quickly being eradicated with employee doctors having comparable salaries and in many cases, better retirement packages. Unfortunately, doctors in all settings now need to spend more time documenting their activities and placing them in the categories required for billing purposes than would be desired by most. Another unfortunate feature of the contemporary medical environment is the high cost of medical malpractice insurance, sometimes topping $200,000 annually for certain specialties.

On the bright side, because of a fantastic basic science enterprise, doctors have never been able to understand diseases and offer better treatments—both medical and surgical—than today. Government-supported basic research combined with the much more expensive industry-supported clinical science studies has led to unprecedented medical treatments. Unfortunately, the expense of these efforts and the need to attract investment in new drug opportunities, most of which fail, result in very high costs for the newest drugs. However, competition has resulted in the vast majority of drugs being relatively inexpensive— in the United States 90% of drugs are generic. Overall, today doctors practice in an environment that allows them tremendous opportunity to help their patients and the public. However, health care in the U.S. is costly and suffers from the problems of decentralized systems. Other countries suffer the frustrations of a single system.

CHAPTER **16**

SOME OTHER CONSIDERATIONS

What percentage of United States doctors are foreign-born and trained?

What are the upsides and downsides of care in teaching hospitals?

Selecting Your Doctor

There is and always has been a great degree of randomness in people's selection of their physicians. Choices are obviously limited by location and by finance. Regardless of the prevailing health-care system, most people will have doctors based on availability and convenience rather than on a deliberate choice. Nevertheless, a key factor in continuing with or selecting a physician is your comfort level with the doctor's personality and style. Consider asking yourself the following questions:

- Can I easily understand what the doctor says?
- Is the doctor too directive or paternalistic? Or perhaps, too nondirective?
- Is the doctor's visit too brief or perhaps too drawn out?
- Is the doctor open to questions?
- Are the doctor's explanations too filled with jargon or not technical enough?
- Am I comfortable with the doctor's dress and manner?

A good fit is important to minimize doubts and maximize the therapeutic effect of the doctor and the treatments. When you sense that the doctor is not a good fit for you, change doctors if possible. Most systems make it possible to change without a direct encounter with the current doctor.

Foreign-Trained Doctors

About 25 percent of US doctors are foreign-born and trained. They are known as non-US Foreign Medical Graduates (FMG). In addition, many native-born US doctors have trained in medicine outside of the US. Many FMGs will have taken post-medical-school training in the US. FMGs account for a disproportionately high number of US general physicians and make up a rather high percentage of the physicians in rural America. All of them have had to pass numerous tests and rigorous selection systems both for US training and to obtain US state medical licenses. As such, patients can have a high level of confidence in their abilities, especially with those FMGs who are providing highly technical services or consultant services. In some cases, FMGs may have accents that are difficult for patients to quickly and fully understand and might also have a value system that is slightly different than is customary for the region. These limitations may not be too important when the FMG is providing highly technical or consultatory service. However, when serving as a patient's generalist, they could be important. For example, for patients with age related hearing impairment or diminished acuity.

Teaching Hospitals

The phrase "teaching hospitals" encompasses both hospitals and outpatient facilities that are part of or affiliated with a medical school and in some cases schools of allied health sciences, such as nursing and pharmacy schools. Being a patient at a teaching hospital or university most often means that your care may be given, participated in, or observed by doctors or students at varying levels of training. Many people view this as undesirable and avoid teaching hospitals. In addition, in teaching hospitals your care may feel fragmented even producing real confusion as to who is actually your doctor. While this attitude is understandable, the upside or favorable side of having training doctors involved is that they offer another brain and set of eyes on your circumstances and help ensure that your attending or main physician is aware that their activities and decisions are being watched and studied.

In addition, university doctors will almost always be familiar with the most up-to-date information and thinking and will often have technologies not yet widely available. The upside of teaching centers should be considered when you are physically near enough to comfortably access care at a teaching center or when your care seems inadequate and you want other options.

Game Changing Technologies

As noted earlier, doctors are the interface (learned intermediaries) between new technologies and patients. Certain technologies, such as standardized electronic medical records used and accessible by all health care systems and wearable or implanted health monitors will broadly impact all of health care. Patients, even now, will benefit themselves by taking responsibility for having their electronic records. Similarly, patients should assume responsibility for providing end-of-life guidance.

Understanding Your Doctors

As noted, it is important that you are comfortable with and have confidence in your doctors. It is in your interest to be certain that your doctors understand you as an individual and toward that end you should endeavor to let your doctor know as much about you and your past and present activities as possible. The "little old ladies" bringing cookies and cakes to their doctor may have been on to something.

Similarly, it is helpful for you to know personal details about your doctor. Perhaps one general idea that is applicable to all doctors is that they do not think of themselves as wealthy or rich. Rather, as people who are well paid. Because of time put into their work and education, they believe they are paid appropriately. They generally believe that they do not work for money but rather to help people. The systems doctors are in, the polite and most often grateful patients, the supportive nurses, office assistants, and so forth sustain their belief that they are the good guys, not rich guys.

Made in the USA
Monee, IL
30 October 2024

69008439R10049